Leptin Resistance

Leptin Diet to Control Your Hormones, Get Permanent Weight Loss, Cure Obesity and Live Healthy

LELA GIBSON

CONTENTS

Introduction

I want to thank you and congratulate you for buying the book, *"Leptin Resistance: Leptin Diet to Control Your Hormones, Get Permanent Weight Loss, Cure Obesity and Live Healthy"*.

This book has lots of actionable information on how to fight leptin resistance to control your hormones and ultimately bring about lasting weight loss and health.

Are you addicted to food? Are you also constantly gaining weight you cannot seem to lose no matter what you try? If yes, chances are you are leptin resistant. The solution to this problem lies within the Leptin Diet, a diet designed to reset your leptin levels or sensitivity.

The interesting thing about the Leptin Diet is that it is neither a pleasure depriving diet nor a starvation routine camouflaged diet. It is a diet centered on what foods to eat and when to eat them.

This book shall teach you everything you need to know about using food to reset and normalize your leptin sensitivity, control the synthesis of hormones within the body, how by resting your leptin levels, you can start losing weight and keep it at bay forever, and above all, how to live a healthy life free from obesity and its deathly hollows. Let's begin.

Thanks again for buying this book. I hope you enjoy it!

Before we can get to a point of discussing how to follow the Leptin Diet to lose weight and keep it off, it is important that we start by building an understanding of what leptin is and the role it plays in the body..

Understanding Leptin and Its Function within the Body

What Is Leptin And What Is Its Function In The Body?

Leptin, usually referred to as the satiety or starvation hormone, is a hormone secreted from stored fat cells of the white adipose tissues. This means the amount of leptin in your bloodstream is directly proportionate to your total body fat. In simple terms, the higher your body fat, the greater the amount of leptin you produce. Its primary target is the hypothalamus, the part of the brain in control of when and how much you should eat.

Once released from the adipose tissue, Leptin circulates in the bloodstream and ends up in the brain. Its main function is to tell the brain you have enough energy stored in your fat reserves and therefore, your body can start normal metabolic processes. In simple terms, leptin is the medium through which your fat stores speak to your brain to let it know how much energy is available and what the body can do with it.

When it comes to understanding your feelings of hunger and satiety, Leptin is the most important hormone. When produced in high quantities, it signals the brain to tell you that you are full and you should stop eating. When its level drops, you start feeling hungry and you begin craving food. This happens because it stimulates receptors in your brain's hypothalamus. Leptin molecules attach themselves to receptors in this part of your brain and the hypothalamus reacts by releasing appetite-suppressing or supporting chemicals.

Low leptin levels stimulate the hypothalamus to produce some chemicals namely NPY (neuropeptide Y) and anandamide, both of which are strong feeding stimulants and they drive up your hunger levels. On the contrary, high leptin levels also stimulate the hypothalamus to produce another chemical called alpha-MSH (alpha-Melanocyte stimulating hormone), an appetite suppressant that makes you feel satiated such that you no longer feel like eating.

Each person has a genetically set level of leptin threshold. Whenever your leptin levels go above that threshold, your brain detects you have ample energy to expend and your body can therefore use this energy at a normal rate. When you lose weight rapidly, either by consuming fewer calories or through liposuction (cosmetic procedure/plastic surgery to remove excessive body fat), your body uses some of the stored fat as energy to make up for that deficit. This leads to a decrease in the amounts of leptin produced.

The brain senses that fat stores are low and that you are on the brink of starvation. Consequently, you get hungrier. Your thyroid reduces its output and your metabolic rate plummets. Your body's catabolic hormone activity intensifies and so does your appetite. You then end up abandoning your dieting regime and regaining back all that lost fat mass. This is why crash dieting is ineffective because even when you lose weight rapidly and in a short span of time, low leptin levels will not let you feed less and even if you somehow manage to do so, your metabolic rate will decrease considerably.

Another noteworthy fact is that leptin is more sensitive to starvation than it is to overeating. When you adopt a diet that emphasizes calorie restriction and you manage to lose some fat, leptin levels fall rapidly. On the other hand, if you eat more than you usually do, leptin levels do not rise instantly. Rather, they increase gradually depending on how much food you have eaten.

Even if the above mechanism seems to work perfectly, it can get corrupted and start malfunctioning, something that is likely to bring about lots of other problems. To help you understand that, we will discuss insulin resistance in the next chapter.

How Leptin Resistance Develops

Those who are overweight or obese have more than necessary body fat in their fat cells. Since the fat cells are responsible for secreting leptin in proportion to the amount of body fat, such persons produce very high amounts of leptin. Considering the way in which leptin functions, and given the brain knows that the body has more than enough energy reserves, such people should not actually eat.

The problem however is that with extremely elevated levels of leptin over a prolonged period, the brain gets to a point where it gets 'deaf' to the bombardment of leptin. In that case, it requires more leptin to produce the same satiety effect. This phenomenon is what we call **leptin resistance.** Scientists believe leptin resistance is the major biological abnormality in human obesity.

Leptin resistance occurs when your body experiences continuous overexposure to high levels of leptin to a point where eventually, this overexposure affects your brain's sensitivity to leptin. When your body becomes resistant to leptin, it may require a much higher quantity of leptin before the brain signals the body that you feel full. In this case, if you are obese, while you already have abnormally high amounts of leptin, you are unresponsive to it.

Since the brain is not sensing the presence of leptin, it mistakenly believes the body is going through a period of starvation even though it is evident there are abnormally high stores of fat. Accordingly, the brain reacts by changing the physiology and behavior of the body in a bid to increase fat stores rather than burn them.

How does it do that? Well, the brain keeps your appetite constant and it decreases satiety with eating such that there is no reduction in hunger. The brain also feels that the body needs to conserve energy so you end up feeling lazier and undergo a decrease in resting metabolism. The result is that you eat more, exercise less, and end up gaining weight.

Even when healthy persons with standard BMI index restrict their calorie intake for a couple of meals, studies show that their leptin levels still decrease as expected but they end up experiencing hunger pangs and feeling less energetic because of a reduced rate of metabolism. This happens even when there is no significant change in weight. For that reason, if you wish to lose weight, you ought to allow adequate time for your body to adjust to the new level where it has low levels of leptin.

Note:

You do not have to be overweight to become resistant to leptin. A recent study published in the American journal of Physiology now reveals that high sugar (especially fructose) diets can induce leptin resistance. These sugars impair leptin's ability to cross the blood brain barrier and reach the hypothalamus such that even when leptin levels are high, not enough reaches the brain and therefore, the brain does not signal the body that it is full.

Let's discuss more about what contributes to leptin resistance.

Factors Contributing to Leptin Resistance

As we have discussed in passing, leptin resistance is a condition not confined to the obese. As medical research has discovered, the following factors can lead to leptin resistance:

1: High Fructose Intake

Fructose is a natural simple sugar found in honey, fruits, and vegetables. Food and drink sweeteners such as high fructose corn syrup (HCFS) are also high in fructose. Fructose is also the major constituent of brown sugar, table sugar, agave, maple syrup, and molasses.

A recent research study conducted by scientists from the University of Florida and published in the American Journal of Physiology, Regulatory, Integrative, and Comparative Physiology showed how diets high in fructose caused leptin resistance in rats and how it eventually made them overweight.

For a period of 6 months, the rats, divided into two groups, fed on various diets. The first group fed on a diet free from any fructose while the other group fed on a diet comprised of 60% fructose. When the period was over, researchers tested the leptin levels of rats from both groups.

They discovered that the rats that fed on a 60% fructose diet had developed resistance to leptin. Surprisingly, the same rats also had higher levels of **triglycerides** in their bloodstream. In the other group of fats, there was no significant change in the levels of leptin, insulin, glucose, and cholesterol.

Afterwards, the scientists isolated half the number of rats from each group and they fed them a high fat diet for a fortnight. The rats that were earlier on a 60% fructose diet increased their amount of food consumption and consequently put on more weight than rats that were on a fructose free diet.

From these results, the researchers concluded that diets that combine high amounts of fructose with high amounts of fats and calories worsen the obesity epidemic.

From this study, researchers concluded that fructose affects the leptin pathways in two ways. The first is that on its own, high fructose promptly renders innate the hypothalamus' resistant to leptin. In other words, normal functioning receptors in the hypothalamus seem to become weak and ineffective in the presence of leptin when fructose levels in the blood are high.

Secondly, consumption of fructose results in the body producing tons of triglycerides. Triglycerides block the passage of leptin to the brain. This study shows that triglycerides promote leptin resistance by impairing leptin transport across the BBB (blood brain barrier), which means not enough leptin gets to the receptors in the brain to produce the desired effect.

2: Lectin Consumption

Lectins are a type of protein found in many plant foods. They attach to carbohydrates and other biological structures of a plant, which allows them to cause harm as part of the plant's self-defense mechanism against natural enemies such as fungi and insects.

In general, Lectins are a form of glycan-binding proteins. This means if ingested, they can also attach to carbohydrates in the body. For humans, unfortunately, some of these lectins can cause harm to the body by causing inflammation and leaky gut; they also contribute to leptin resistance.

One type of Lectin called wheat germ agglutinin (WGA) commonly found in some members of the grass family such as wheat, millet, and barley causes leptin resistance by directly binding with the leptin receptor. This then prevents the leptin from binding instead. Leptin failing to bind with leptin receptors adequately describes leptin resistance and this makes Lectins intensifiers of leptin resistance.

Among the plants that contain the highest amounts of Lectins include seeds of the grass family (such as wheat, rye, barley, rice, oats, wheat germ, millet, corn, quinoa, among others), legumes such as soy, lentils, peanuts, and all kinds of dried beans, and members of the nightshade family such as tomatoes, potatoes, eggplants and peppers. Dairy produce may also have traces of this substance especially if it is grain fed rather than pasture fed.

3: Drastic Calorie Restriction

By now, you know that over-dieting restrains the production of leptin. Do not adopt diets that advocate for calorie restriction of less than 1,000 calories because these will cause a drastic and profound reduction in your circulating levels of leptin. This is according to this authoritative study.

Actually, rapid and severe reduction in calorie consumption decreases leptin levels faster than could be explained by body fat losses (and the same is true for binge eating).

Losing weight using the calorie restriction method is extremely difficult because the leaner you become and the more you continue to restrict calories, the more your leptin levels plummet, and the more your appetite and hunger intensifies. If you ask someone who has been using this method of dieting, he or she will tell you that sheer strength of mind can never be stronger than hormonal drive. At the end of the day, your determination will always give way to your hormones.

4: Inadequate Sleep

Sleep is a very important aspect of your health since it helps restore you on a mental, physical, and emotional level. When you sleep well, your body is refreshed and energized. However, when you fail to get adequate sleep, you feel fatigued, irritable, and sluggish throughout the day. The National Sleep Foundation's recommendation is that adults ought to sleep for about 7-9 hours every night. Failure to do so may cause leptin resistance.

In a different study published in the American Heart Association's Epidemiology and Prevention, the researchers examined 17 healthy and young people for 8 nights. Half of those slept normally and the rest slept for 2/3 of their normal sleeping period.

The findings were that the persons who were 'sleep deprived' ate an extra 549 calories every day on average. There were no noticeable changes in activity energy expenditure. Increased caloric consumption without increase in energy expenditure means weight gain, more leptin production, and even constant increase in fat mass.

Tests actually showed that the sleep-deprived subjects had increased leptin levels. If this study had taken longer than those 8 nights, the sleep-deprived subjects would have probably become leptin resistant because of their ever-increasing leptin levels.

5: Insulin Resistance

Repeated insulin spikes, mainly because of high sugar diet, can cause insulin resistance. This is because when high levels of insulin constantly barrage your body, it reaches a point where the cells no longer respond to insulin as they should.

Professor Robert H. Lustig, a pediatric endocrinologist at UCSF Benioff Hospital has reasons to believe insulin resistance plays a key role in causing leptin resistance. Even more importantly, he discovered that when you reduce your insulin levels, you can also improve leptin signaling (the brain's ability to respond to leptin signals), and this can help you stop unhealthy cravings, promote satiety when full and hunger when starving, and more importantly, it can trigger weight loss.

According to his book, Fat Chance, Lustig believes leptin resistance and high sugar diets are the causes of the worldwide epidemic of obesity. Such a diet triggers leptin resistance even when your BMI index is slightly above the standard range. He explains that 1.5 billion obese and overweight persons around the globe suffer from Leptin resistance and he is certain that targeting insulin can help deal with this.

Studies published in his book reveal the roles of insulin and leptin have an intricate entanglement and that they both attach to receptors in the hypothalamus. These two hormones frequently go together because many people have developed both types of resistance.

When you ingest plenty of sugar, the pancreas secretes insulin in copious amounts. Since leptin stimulates biochemical reactions that send satiety signals to the brain, the presence of insulin can cause blockage of these signals and thus no satiety, which means increased cravings and uncontrolled eating of sugars and fatty foods. This amounts to leptin resistance as it blunts the brain's ability to react to leptin signals.

Surprisingly, one of the other leptin functions is to tell the brain to suppress the production of insulin in healthy persons. This happens when leptin dampens your appetite and therefore reduces or stops food consumption. This in turn reduces the body's need to produce more insulin to work on the food already in the system.

When you are insulin resistant (or have high levels of insulin), and when you are leptin resistant, this does not happen. In fact, your insulin levels just keep soaring higher to create a vicious cycle. Lustig explains that the insidious creep of insulin resistance makes your body produce two times the amount of insulin for every teaspoon of sugar you consume as compared to what the body produced 30 years ago.

6: Chronic Inflammation

Fat biology researchers at Harvard Medical School discovered that groups of molecules involved in reducing inflammation also hamper the process of leptin signaling. These molecules also go by SOCS (suppressors of cytokine signaling).

In particular, the body produces SOCS-1, and SOCS-3 in response to inflammation and studies show that they are notorious for causing leptin resistance. They do so by blocking the signals leptin is supposed to deliver to the brain and muscle cells. The body releases these SOCS when the inflammation is because of a sudden injury or invasion of pathogens to contain the situation and avoid further damage to cells and tissues. Levels of SOCS subside when the inflammation abates.

When you are under inflammation, SOCS-1 and SOCS-3 molecules assemble in your hypothalamus and they jam leptin's signals at the internal portion of the leptin receptor such that the message to suppress satiety does not go through. Therefore, SOCS molecules released to counter inflammation are the primary causes of leptin resistance in the brain.

Other causes of Leptin Resistance include:

1. High stress levels

2. Uncontrolled eating /overeating

3. Over-exercising

With all the contributing factors, I know you might be wondering; so what are the signs that you have insulin resistance? That's what we will discuss next.

Leptin Resistance Warning Signs and Symptoms

A person with leptin resistance may have no less than two of the following signs:

1. Continuous weight gain and a voracious appetite

2. Difficulty in losing weight even after exercising regularly and dieting

3. Uncontrolled food cravings for sweet and salty junk foods even after a huge meal

4. Fatigue or having low energy or feeling sluggish

5. Deteriorating complications of hypothyroidism (a condition where your thyroid glands do not produce enough thyroid hormones) such as joint pains, infertility, obesity etc.

6. Cold body temperatures that are less than 36°C or 98°F

7. Slow resting heart rate (below 60), which is a result of poor aerobic conditioning and being overweight or obese

8. Reduced sex drive and infertility

Most of these signs may not necessarily mean you are resistant to leptin; however, it should be a cause for concern if you happen to experience more than 2 of these symptoms. If that is the case, chances are high that you might be leptin resistant and you should visit a doctor for serum blood testing.

The doctor may review your history of illness and assess your symptoms before taking a blood sample from a vein on your arm for further tests to determine your leptin levels. Depending on how the results pan out, the doctor can make a diagnosis or recommend further tests because leptin levels may vary from one day to another.

The doctor can advise you to visit again to check leptin levels for diagnosis. The optimum serum-leptin level should be below 10-12. If it is greater than that and you are no less than 9 kgs (20 pounds) overweight, you may be leptin resistant.

The question you might now be having is; so how can you fight leptin resistance? Well, you do that by following the Leptin Diet. In the next chapter, we will discuss 5 rules of the Leptin Diet.

The 5-Rules of the Leptin Diet

Below are the 5 guidelines that form the basis of the Leptin Diet. Much emphasis is on the quality and timing of your food. The diet seeks to give you more energy from less food and more importantly, help you regain control over your leptin sensitivity.

When adopting this diet, you can still eat foods you enjoy as long as they do not contribute to leptin resistance. These principles apply to everyone regardless of age, sex, weight, or even otherwise. The Leptin Diet is a long-term diet that can fit (seamlessly so) into your lifestyle and in the process, help you live happily and healthfully.

1st Rule: Consume the Right Amounts of Macronutrients

The type of macronutrient you eat sends a specific message to your body. These messages are what alter the levels of your hormones. With that said, you have to make sure you influence and send the right messages to your body with the kind of foods you eat.

For example, when you eat proteins, you increase mTOR (the mechanistic target of rapamycin), a central metabolism regulator that promotes growth. If you eat carbohydrates (especially in excessive amounts), you increase insulin levels and end up sending a signal for growth. Only fats do not send any growth signals.

Most people have grown to believe that only a diet comprised of just enough carbohydrates can help you lower levels of insulin and leptin. What most people do not know is that eating too much protein even as you lower you lower your carb intake still brings the opposite of the desired effect.

Therefore, your diet should consist of high fats, medium proteins, and carbohydrates. Your proteins still need to be adequate to ensure you maintain your muscle mass. Carbohydrates should also be just enough to maintain healthy insulin levels and energy levels.

Dr. Westin Childs, a doctor who specializes in weight loss by striking the right hormonal balance recommends the ratio of fats to carbs to proteins be **60:20:20** respectively, which you can then slightly alter with time as your leptin resistance begins to ease.

This means you should derive 60% of your total calories from high quality and healthy sources of fat. 20% percent of your calories should be from high quality carbohydrates and the remaining 20% should come from high quality organic sources of protein. This kind of diet will keep your insulin and mTOR at optimum levels.

2nd Rule: Only Eat Three Times a Day

Maintain a 4-6 hour gap between meals and do not snack. Each time you snack, you are having an extra meal. Your body's metabolism system cannot deal with continuous eating. A habit of snacking every now and then confuses your metabolism and you increase the amount of calories you consume every day, which as you may guess, leads to weight gain.

It is important that you give your body some 'breathing' space between meals; your body uses this time to clear the remaining triglyceride fat blobs from your blood stream. If you do not allow your body enough time to clear these, they will end up clogging your leptin receptors in the hypothalamus, which will lead to leptin resistance.

Snacking between meals is one of the greatest lies of our generation. We have heard that snacking stokes up your metabolism and helps you maintain blood sugar at optimum levels. Most of us believe this lie. But the truth is; when you keep snacking, you consume more calories, which flick on the powerful switches that cause leptin dysfunction. The 'snack lie' has only inflated the obesity epidemic.

The only snack you should have between meals should come from your liver. This helps your body clear triglycerides naturally. These triglycerides not only block the leptin receptors in the brain, they also travel to various organs such as the stomach, hips, and thighs. That is why it is imperative that you allow the body enough time to break them down and clear them from your system. You can only achieve that by giving your body a period of 4-6 hours between meals.

For leptin to be effective, you need to clear your circulatory highways of extra fat and even the fat stored around other areas of your body.

3rd Rule: Never Eat After Dinner

Let dinner be the last meal of the day: **PERIOD!** Make sure you leave a gap of 3 hours (minimum) between dinner and going to bed. Never go to bed on a full stomach. Also, make sure you maintain 11-12 hours between dinner and breakfast. If you snack in the middle of the night, or sleep immediately after dinner, chances are high that every single calorie you have eaten will go into storage as body fat.

Some of our bodies have become accustomed to having midnight snacks as a way of de-stressing or relaxing before going back to sleep again. Most people struggle to fall back into slumber if they do not sleepily wobble to the refrigerator in the dead of night.

Leptin levels rise and fall at a regular rhythm that follows a 24-hour pattern. Researchers in this field have observed that levels of leptin peak at the evening hours. This happens so that the body may undergo nighttime self-repair and recovery. Leptin is the hormone that coordinates the timing and production of hormone melatonin, the hormone that allows for entrainment (synchronization) of the circadian rhythm, metabolism, and body rejuvenation while sleeping. However, all this will happen if you do not eat or snack at all after dinner.

4th Rule: Avoid Large Meals

If you have successfully stopped snacking and you are now eating 3 meals a day, the next thing you should be aware of is a need to overcompensate your usual eating habits with large meal servings. If that is the case, you are doing more harm than good since you are overfeeding and giving your body too much energy at once.

To solve this, you need to eat small portions and do so slowly because the satiety signal usually comes between 10 and 20 minutes into your meal. When you eat slowly, you give your body enough time to process the amount of food you have eaten and then tell you to stop when you are full.

It is important to listen to your internal cues and stop eating when you feel full to avoid overeating. This is what most non-obese people do: they stop when they get the satiety signal. For people who struggle with weight issues however, food portion size largely depends on what is available. This is what we often refer to as the 'see food diet' because what you see is what you eat, no matter how big it is.

Turn away from this habit because all it will do is lead to even more resistance and entrapment into obesity where it will be taking longer for you to feel full meaning you will keep eating more.

5th Rule: Make High Quality Proteins Part of Your Breakfast

Your breakfast should consist of a moderate amount of proteins every day, less at lunchtime and if possible, you should not have any for dinner to make sure you do not exceed the daily 20% limit of calories from proteins. Oddly enough, for most people, dinner is usually the largest meal of the day. However, if you are struggling with food cravings, low energy, and weight issues, you should opt to focus on breakfast. Having a protein rich breakfast will boost your metabolism and keep you energized for long periods.

The advantage with this kind of breakfast is that it increases your metabolism by 30% for a period of around 12 hours. This is equivalent to burning calories by jogging for 2 or 3 miles. A high quality carb breakfast comprising of cereal, pancakes, bagels, or waffles coupled with a little amount of protein cannot improve your metabolism to above 4%. For some people, a higher carbohydrate breakfast seems to make their metabolism run just fine, but that does not work quite well for someone struggling with weight.

A high protein breakfast can include foods such as eggs and tomatoes, cottage, cheddar or ricotta cheese, fish, along with a serving of healthy dose of fats like a spoon of coconut oil or nuts and some carbs, fruit or salad dressing. Other rich sources of protein include soymilk, skim milk, Greek yogurt, wheat meat, peanut butter, and mozzarella and pumpkin seeds among others.

With that in mind, the tips in the next chapter will help sustain you throughout your journey as you follow the Leptin Diet.

Tips for Reversing Leptin Resistance

While everything we have discussed thus far shall help you reverse leptin resistance, the following tips will rocket fuel your journey:

1: Exercise Regularly but Do Not Over-Train

Regular exercise helps burn calories; it can also help you regain your leptin sensitivity and keep you from developing leptin resistance. A study published in the open access journal PLoS Biology in August 2010 showed how exercise increased IL-6 and IL-10 protein levels in the hypothalamus of overweight rats. Researchers also discovered that both IL-6 and IL-10 molecules increase the sensitivity of leptin and insulin.

You can try doing low intensity exercises like walking, jogging, cycling, dancing, swimming, skipping rope, sport, and even some household chores. 20 to 30 minutes of physical activity per day is enough to up your fitness levels. The number of activities you can do to increase your heart rate is in plenty. If you are not very physically fit, you can start slowly and then gradually work your way up as you increase the frequency and intensity.

Do not forget that too much of everything is dangerous. Many people with leptin resistance make the mistake of overtraining so they can lose more weight in a short span of time.

What they do not know is that in doing so, they make it even the more difficult to shed a few pounds and here is why.

Pushing your training regimen beyond the set limit raises your cortisol levels because of the stress you exert on your body. High cortisol levels can alter your insulin levels and consequently, make weight loss difficult to achieve.

2: Cold Therapy/Exposure

Yes, you read that right. If you did not know, exposing yourself to cold temperatures has plenty of health benefits. It can aid in speedy recovery from injury, reduce pain threshold, improve quality of sleep, bone health, immune system, lifespan etc., and more importantly, it helps you lose weight.

Studies show that leptin receptors are more efficient when you expose yourself to cold temperatures. Therefore, cold therapy can reverse insulin resistance by increasing leptin sensitivity.

Cold therapy is actually very simple and you can do it from the comfort of your home by turning down the house's thermostat. You can also bath in a bathtub filled with cold water or you can swim in cold water. You can also use crycotherapy iceboxes mostly used in the field of sports medicine.

The tips above will certainly skyrocket the efficiency with which you see the benefits of leptin resistance.

Sample Leptin Diet Meal Plan (With Recipes)

On the Leptin diet, having many meals a day or snacking between meals is discouraged; three main meals are enough, typically breakfast, lunch and dinner- no dessert. Below is a basic example of how your meal plan should look like:

Breakfast
Brown Bread and Boiled Eggs

Servings: 1

Ingredients

2 eggs

Flaky sea salt, e.g. Maldon

¼ English cucumber- sliced

2 slices pumpernickel bread- cut in half (Recipe below)

2 tablespoons butter or cream cheese- softened

Instructions

Add eggs to a medium heavy saucepan and pour in water up to 1 ½ inches. Bring to a boil then remove pan from heat right away.

Cover and let it stand for about 10 minutes after which place the eggs in a bowl of ice water to cool.

Crack the eggshells and peel off shell.

Spread butter on your bread and serve with the cucumber and eggs seasoned with sea salt.

Enjoy!

Note:

For the Pumpernickel Bread (makes 2 small round loaves):

Ingredients

3 cups bread flour

4 teaspoons salt

2 tablespoons caraway seed

2 ¾ cups rye flour

1 ½ tablespoons active dry yeast

1 ½ cups warm water

½ cup molasses

2 tablespoons shortening

Instructions

Add yeast and warm water to a large bowl and stir until yeast dissolves.

Add the shortening, molasses, rye flour, salt and caraway seeds and stir.

Add 2 cups of bread flour and mix then slowly add the rest of the bread flour until you get dough good enough for kneading.

Put the dough onto a floured board, knead for around 5 minutes and if it is too sticky, knead in some bread flour 1 tablespoon at a time.

Put the dough into a greased bowl and flip it over to grease the top lightly.

Cover using a plastic wrap or a clean kitchen towel for about an hour (or until double in size) to allow the dough to rise in a warm place.

After an hour, pat down the dough, cover again and let it rise for 45 more minutes.

Pat the dough again and turn it out onto a surface or board that is lightly floured and knead for a little while.

Cut the dough into 2 even portions and shape each half into a small and round loaf.

Use oil to grease a baking sheet and sprinkle some cornmeal on it (if desired).

Place both loaves on the baking sheet, cover and allow the dough to rise until double in size (about 45 minutes).

Bake both round loaves in the oven at 375 degrees F for about 35 minutes or until when tapped, the bread feels hollow.

Remove from the oven and let the bread cool on a rack. You can wrap the loaves in plastic or freeze for later.

Lunch
Coconut Rice with Grilled Shrimp

Servings: 6

Ingredients

2 peeled and diced Roma tomatoes

1 teaspoon fresh ginger, minced

6 cloves of garlic

1 cup organic low fat vanilla yogurt

1 ¾ cups of basmati rice

2 red or yellow peppers, diced

½ cup chopped parsley

2 tablespoons olive oil

3 cups of water

1 white onion, diced

¼ cup unsweetened, grated coconut

Salt and pepper to taste

1 lb. shrimp (16-20 count)- peeled and deveined

Instructions

Soak 6 wooden skewers in water for about 20 to 30 minutes.

Add olive oil to a large saucepan (fitted with a lid) and heat over medium high heat.

Toss in the peppers and onion and cook for 5 minutes until the onion turns translucent.

Add the garlic and ginger and cook as you stir until fragrant.

Toss in the coconut and tomatoes and mix everything well and cook for 5 more minutes.

Add in the rice and cook as you stir continuously for 2 minutes until lightly browned.

Add water and stir to combine then bring to a boil. Reduce the heat to low for a steady simmer. Cover and simmer for about 15 to 20 minutes then remove from heat.

Temper the yogurt by adding it to a small bowl and adding some of the rice mixture then stirring.

Gradually add the rice mixture as you stir until the yogurt is warmed all the way through.

Add all of the bowl contents to the rice mixture together with the parsley, salt and pepper to taste then fold together to combine.

Thread around 4 shrimp for each skewer through the head and tail and grill for 1 to 2 minutes on each side over medium heat (until the shrimp is white in the center).

Serve the coconut rice with the shrimp. Enjoy!

Dinner
Healthy Jambalaya Soup

Servings: 6

Ingredients

250g long grain rice (cooked)

1 large red pepper, deseeded and chopped finely

1 large green pepper, deseeded and chopped finely

2 garlic cloves

25g bunch parsley, leaves chopped roughly

1 onion, halved and finely sliced

1 bay leaf

1.25 liters chicken stock

2½ teaspoons sweet smoked paprika

350g sausages, half smoked half plain, sliced

220g raw shell-on prawns

500g tomato passata

3 sprigs thyme

1 tablespoon oil

1 large celery stalk, chopped

1-3 green and red chilies, sliced

1-2 teaspoons chili powder

Instructions

Heat half of the oil in a pan and add in the celery and onions. Cook for 5 minutes and then add the chili and garlic. Lower the heat and cook for 5 more minutes.

Add in the thyme, spices and bay leaf, mix well then pour in the stock and passata. Bring to a boil and cover loosely. Let it simmer for about 20 minutes.

Heat the remaining oil in a pan and add in the sausage to fry. Drain on kitchen towel when done then add it to the pot together with the peppers and prawn and heat until cooked.

Add in the hot rice, season and sprinkle some parsley on top.

Snack
Lemon-Apple Smoothie

Servings: 1

Ingredients

½ cup water

1 packet stevia

½ teaspoon ground cinnamon

1 whole carrot

Juice of lemon

1 tablespoon almond butter

1 cup kale, washed

1 cup almond milk

3 dates

1 granny smith apple

Instructions

Was all the veggies then peel and chop the carrots.

Take out the seeds from the apple and chop it.

Toss in the chopped apple and all other ingredients into the blender and blend until smooth.

Serve and enjoy.

I need your help...

We have come to the end of the book. Thank you for reading and congratulations for reading until the end.

It is important to keep in mind that research on leptin and leptin resistance is still in its formative stages. The hormone is a recent discovery (discovered in 1994), and much of what we now know comes from animal studies, and very few from clinical trials involving humans. One thing is for sure though; there is no doubt that the discovery of leptin has continued to revolutionize the health sector especially in regards to curing obesity, the worldwide epidemic.

Overcoming leptin resistance does not have to be a tedious endeavor. With a few key lifestyle and dietary changes, you can regain control over proper leptin function in your body and transform your road to great health from a potholed path to a super highway.

Finally, if you enjoyed this book, would you be kind enough to leave a review for this book on Amazon?

Pleave a review for this book on Amazon!

Thank you and good luck!

Preview Of 'Anti-Inflammatory Diet Guide'

Effects Of Inflammation

Inflammation is the biological response your body goes into when dealing with harmful stimuli such as irritants, pathogens or even damaged cells. It is a self-protection mechanism that allows your body to begin the healing process. The 'hotness' or 'inflammation' you feel after you cut yourself or injure yourself is the result of your body working hard to heal itself. But what happens when your body experiences 'too much' inflammation?

A little inflammation is not a bad thing. In fact, when it happens, you should rejoice in knowing that your body is working tirelessly to correct the situation. However, like most good things, inflammation can get out of hand. When this happens, you may experience various health complications such as:

Weight Gain

Every day, thousands of people try to lose weight to no avail. They complain that they've tried out various diets but somehow none seem to be working. If they do find something that works, sooner than later, they are back to gaining the weight they thought they'd lost. This is because they neglect to look into inflammation as the cause for their weight gain. Inflammation contributes to weight gain in various ways. These include:

- If inflammation happens in the brain, it interferes with the functioning of the hypothalamus and this in turn increases your appetite and slows down your metabolism. When this happens, you will be eating a lot but burning up less energy, which leads to weight gain.

- Gut inflammation leads to leptin and insulin resistance. Leptin is the satiety hormone that tells your brain when you have had enough. When suffering from leptin resistance, you just eat and eat some more before leptin can communicate that you have had enough, which leads to weight gain. Another thing that gut inflammation does is to increase intestinal permeability. When this happens, more toxins will be able to permeate your bloodstream. Usually toxins are stored in fat cells to remove them from circulation. The more toxins you have, the more the fat cells expand to accommodate the more toxins leading to weight gain.

- Inflammation in the endocrine system suppresses adrenal and thyroid function. One of the main functions of the adrenal gland is to burn fat. Therefore, when you suppress the functioning of the adrenal gland, you are unable to burn fat, as you should leading to weight gain.

As you have read, inflammation is bad for you if you want to maintain the ideal weight.

Metabolic Syndrome

Metabolic syndrome refers to a group/cluster of lifestyle-related diseases including cardiovascular disease and obesity. They are clustered together because all of these diseases are linked to metabolic dysfunction. Markers of metabolic dysfunction include:

- Central obesity – this is excessive tummy fat

- Hyperinsulinaemia – this refers to ongoing high levels of insulin

- Insulin resistance –your body loses sensitivity to insulin (you need more insulin to manage your blood sugar levels)

But the question is how these three factors are connected. Well, when on a diet high in carbohydrates, your blood sugar levels increase leading to high insulin levels to help blood cells absorb the glucose and thus manage your blood sugar levels. When you have high insulin levels, the production of cytokines (which are pro-inflammatory) increases and in turn this causes inflammation especially in predisposed persons. Once inflammation increases, it brings with it an increase in the production of free radicals. Free radicals affect cellular functions and one of those functions just happens to be insulin sensitivity. This is why chroni low-grade inflammation is linked to all three markers; that is, raised insulin levels, obesity and decreased insulin sensitivity.

Chronic Fatigue

Many people suffering from chronic fatigue have been told that the disease 'is all in their minds'. Fortunately, in recent years more researchers have began looking into the association of chronic fatigue and inflammation. This is mainly because the two possess many similar symptoms including muscular pain and tenderness, sore throat, joint pain, swollen lymph nodes and sore throat.

As you know, inflammation is the way your body reacts to foreign particles. When you have symptoms of inflammation, it is safe to say that your body is fighting something even if that something is not yet known. This is why researchers link an overactive immune system to chronic fatigue.

Another thing that associates chronic fatigue with inflammation is the lack of cortisol in patients suffering from chronic fatigue. Cortisol is known to suppress inflammation. Thus, if your body has a cortisol deficiency, it will not be able to suppress inflammation and this will worsen symptoms of chronic fatigue. A dietary change often helps people suffering from chronic fatigue.

Some types of arthritis

When you hear the name arthritis, you automatically associate it with pain. Well, it is no coincidence since arthritis refers to inflammation in joints. When your joints experience inflammation, you will feel pain. The types of arthritis that have been linked to inflammation include:

- Gouty arthritis

- Rheumatoid arthritis

- Psoriatic arthritis

- Systematic lupus erythematosus

When you suffer from these types of arthritis, you may experience inflammation symptoms such as redness, joint stiffness, swelling of the joints, pain in the joints and loss of joint function.

It is important to note that inflammation does not have to be painful for it to be present. This is because many organs in your body just don't have enough pain-sensitive areas for you to feel that inflammatory sensation. This means that you can suffer from chronic inflammation over time without knowing, only for you to experience the effects of inflammation.

It is also important to note that various things can cause inflammation including:

- Processed foods high in sugar and unhealthy fats

- Omega-6 fats (and not enough Omega-3 fatty acids)

- Sleep deprivation

- Chronic stress

- Smoking

- Pollution

- Environmental chemicals

- Lack of exercise

Thus, chances are, if you experience any of the above things, you may be suffering from inflammation whether or not you experience pain.

The first thing you should do once you notice that you suffer from inflammation is not to reach for drugs because drugs just address the symptoms and not the root cause but rather to make some lifestyle changes. This is because most of the causes of inflammation can be addressed by making lifestyle changes like exercising more, reducing exposure to pollutants, not smoking and dietary changes.

In this book, we will focus on addressing inflammation by adopting an anti-inflammatory diet. Let us learn more about anti-inflammatory diet in the next chapter.

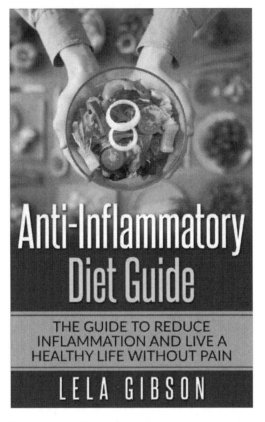

Check out the rest of Anti-Inflammatory Diet Guide on Amazon Or go to: http://amzn.to/2qKTSPa

Check Out My Other Books

Below you'll find some of my other popular books that are popular on Amazon and Kindle as well.

Alternatively, you can visit my author page on Amazon to see other work done by me.

Belly Diet: The Zero Belly Diet Step-By-Step Guide Which Help You To Loose Your Belly And Enjoy Your Flat Belly

Anti-Inflammatory Diet Guide: The Guide To Reduce Inflammation And Live A Healthy Life Without Pain

Negative Calorie Diet: Cookbook & Guide Which Will Help You To Burn Body Fat, Lose Weight And Live Healthy

Clean Eating: Cookbook And Guide To Restore Your Body's Natural Balance And Eat Healthy

Dash Diet: Cookbook For Weight Loss With Action Plan And Easy Recipes

Freedom: How To Make Money Online And Become Financially Free By Creating Passive Income

Weight Loss: 20 Easy And Fast Diet Tips For Losing Weight – An Easy-To-Follow Weight Loss Guide

Smart Fat: Cookbook With Fat Meals Which Help You To Lose Weight, Get Healthy And Improve Brain Function

Made in the USA
Monee, IL
09 June 2021